Khaoula Sibbou
Yassine Smiti
Chat Latifa

Discoid meniscus in children

Khaoula Sibbou
Yassine Smiti
Chat Latifa

Discoid meniscus in children

Use of magnetic resonance imaging in the diagnosis of discoid meniscus

ScienciaScripts

Imprint
Any brand names and product names mentioned in this book are subject to trademark, brand or patent protection and are trademarks or registered trademarks of their respective holders. The use of brand names, product names, common names, trade names, product descriptions etc. even without a particular marking in this work is in no way to be construed to mean that such names may be regarded as unrestricted in respect of trademark and brand protection legislation and could thus be used by anyone.

Cover image: www.ingimage.com

This book is a translation from the original published under ISBN 978-620-2-54801-4.

Publisher:
Sciencia Scripts
is a trademark of
International Book Market Service Ltd., member of OmniScriptum Publishing Group
17 Meldrum Street, Beau Bassin 71504, Mauritius
Printed at: see last page
ISBN: 978-620-3-12756-0

DISCOID MENISCUS IN CHILDREN

Summary

Anatomical reminder of the meniscus 3

A- Medial meniscus : 3

B- Lateral meniscus :... 4

Physiological reminder of the meniscus 5

1.   Cell type... 5

2.   Extracellular matrix 5

Imaging of meniscal lesions [11]... 11

3D Isotropy Turbo Spin-Echo MRI (3D Isotropy Turbo Spin-Echo MRI)

.... 22

The discoid meniscus 23

List of figures 35

References... 36

Anatomical reminder of the meniscus

The meniscal bodies are semilunar fibrocartilages interposed between the femoral condyles and the tibial plateaus. They not only improve the congruence of the joint surfaces, but also induce the "wedge" effect between these two bony elements, and due to their anatomical shape are an important element of knee stabilization. They appear very early in fetal life [1]. These fibrous cartilages are well vascularized at the beginning, but this vascularization progressively decreases with age. Towards the end of puberty, the axial part of the menisci is avascular. Only the peripheral edge remains vascularized [2].

A- Medial meniscus :

It is semi-circular in shape. Its anterior part is much wider than the posterior part. This meniscus is the most stable. Its anterior part is firmly attached in front of the tibial insertion of the anterior cruciate ligament (ACL). This anterior part is connected to the anterior part of the lateral meniscus via the transverse ligament, a dense structure 2 mm in diameter. The posterior part of the medial meniscus is vigorously hooked behind the tibial spine. Its peripheral part is perfectly attached to the capsule along its entire length. In its middle part, the medial meniscus is very well attached to the deep bundle of the medial collateral ligament (LLI) with a reinforcement femoral called the menisco-femoral ligament and a tibial reinforcement called the menisco-tibial ligament. Behind the LLI, the meniscus is attached to the postero-oblique ligament at its tibial part.

B- Lateral meniscus :

It is circular in shape. From front to back, its width is identical. On the other hand, the frequency of shape abnormalities is much higher than in the medial meniscus (1 to 15%), ranging from an increase in the volume of one part of the meniscus to the discoid meniscus. The means of fixation of the lateral meniscus are there. The anterior part is fixed just anteriorly to the tibial spine and posteriorly to the foot of the ACL with which it shares fibrous connections. There is no anatomical relationship with the lateral collateral ligament and/or popliteal tendon. The posterior part of the lateral meniscus has a peculiarity: it is inserted between the insertion of the Humphrey and Wrisberg menisco-femoral ligament, which contributes to its stability. These two ligaments are present in 71% of cases. Both the popliteal muscle and the arcuate popliteal ligament are intimately inserted in the posterior part of the lateral meniscus.

The internal meniscus has a much more limited play than the external meniscus, which induces in the internal compartment an anteroposterior displacement limited to 1 cm during flexion, while in the external compartment it can be as much as 2.5 cm. This contributes to cartilage degeneration after meniscectomy, especially external meniscectomy.

Physiological reminder of the meniscus

I- Functional structure

1. Cell type

The meniscus is a fibrocartilage containing a cell population called fibrochondroblasts, stabilized in an extracellular matrix. These fibrochondroblasts can be optionally specified as fibroblasts or chondrocytes depending on their location on the surface or deep within the meniscal bodies.

2. Extracellular matrix

The extracellular matrix consists of water (75%) and solid material ($\pm\,25\%$). It is mainly collagen, proteoglycans and non-collagenous proteins.

- Collagen

There are at least four types of collagens that can be found in the human adult meniscus. We find predominantly type I (90%), but also types II, V and VI for less than 1 to 2%. The electrophoresis study also suggests the presence of a type III collagen [3]. In menisci, type I collagen is found in bundles [4]. These bundles are arranged according to their location (in depth or on the surface).

The superficial collagen bundles are essentially radially oriented, which guarantees a symmetrical load distributed over the entire meniscus surface.

In order to protect the circumferential stress, the deep collagen fibers have a longitudinal orientation. These bundles run parallel to the meniscal edge, have a diameter of 50 to 150 pm, and are profiled from anterior to posterior and thus participate in the fixation of the meniscus in its anterior and posterior horn. This structure increases the resistance to expulsion of the meniscus under load. Some radially oriented fibers are also found in the deep structure of the meniscus. The fact that these radially oriented bundles are unevenly distributed in an uneven faggle among the deep bundles will promote the degeneration of the meniscal body. The quality of this assembly, as well as the wedge shape of the meniscus contribute to this important function of the meniscus as a shock absorber in the knee.

<u>- Proteoglycans</u>

Proteoglycans constitute a very important structure in the extracellular matrix of the meniscus.

They are fixed in the scaffolding of the collagen fibers. Because of their construction, and fixed in the collagen matrix, these proteoglycans can resist very high compressive forces.

This structure is hydrophilic. Proteoglycans represent a heterogeneous group of glycosaminoglycan chains attached to a core protein. This hydrophilic capacity in an aqueous medium is explained by the sulfate group in their chemical composition. These data explain meniscal turgidity.

- <u>Collagen/proteoglycan/water interaction</u>

Proteoglycans gather, fixed in the structure of collagen fibers. These aggregates are attached to the hyaluronic acid chain. The whole is stabilized by a connecting protein. The electron microscopy study demonstrates very clearly these interactions between collagen and proteoglycans and proteoglycans/proteoglycans.

This whole connection explains the resistance to compressive, distraction and shear forces [5].

- ## Cartilage and meniscal elasticity

The bearing cartilage of the femur and tibia also shows proteoglycan/collagen interactions. In the exercise of axial forces, the repetition of compression and decompression during walking induces a current that leads to the self-lubrication and nutrition of these surfaces. This lubrication film reduces friction. In the axial load the viscoelasticity of the cartilage/meniscus complex increases the bearing surface and thus decreases the load per unit area.

II - <u>Meniscal behaviour</u>

It must be studied in compression, shear and tension.

a- Compression forces

Due to its compressive rigidity and extremely low permeability rate, the meniscus has an extremely efficient structure in the distribution of the load. These elements allow deformation under compression. The study of this behavior has shown that the meniscus reacts anisotropically under compression [6].

b- Shear forces

The study of these forces suggests that the meniscus must withstand high shear forces under normal operating conditions [7]. These forces progressively break the superficial radial fibers but also the deep radial fibers, thus giving rise to the degenerative image of the aged meniscus.

c- Forces in tension

It is clear that resistance to tensile forces depends on the presence and orientation of collagen fibers. Circumferential fibers predominate. The study of bovine menisci shows a tenfold increase in stiffness when evaluated parallel to the collagen bundles versus values measured at right angles.
The difference is even greater when comparing the superficial collagen structure to the deep collagen structure. The resistance to tensile forces is

much lower at the surface due to the net orientation of the collagen fibers.

In addition, the middle meniscus segment is much less resistant to circumferential forces when compared with the anterior and posterior horns. All this is due to the concentration and alignment of the collagen fibers, and all this suggests that the resistance to circumferential tensile stress depends on the ultrastructure of the collagen fibers and therefore on intermolecular interactions. This has a clinical consequence. Horizontal meniscus fractures could be caused by shear forces where the presence of radial fibers in the meniscal body is not in number [8].

III- Functional role of menisci

1- Function on load

The occurrence of degenerative cartilage damage after meniscectomy clearly suggests that menisci play an important role in the transmission of loads in the knee.

In the absence of a load, the contact between the femur and tibia is essentially through the meniscal surface. Only 10% of the load-bearing cartilage is in contact in this situation, and then essentially in the posteromedial part of the tibial plateau. In contrast, the load-bearing cartilage is distributed equally well between the meniscus and the cartilage [9].

2- Damper function

Due to their visco-elastic constitution, menisci attenuate the shock in the loads of walking.

3- Joint stabilizer function

Meniscectomy associated with ligament rupture, particularly in the anterior cruciate ligament, increases knee laxity [10].

4- Lubrication function

Knee joint lubrication is elastohydrodynamic in nature [3]. Since load-bearing surfaces can be deformed under hydrodynamic conditions, the term elastohydrodynamics describes the biological function of the meniscal body in an elegant fagon. Since the articular cartilage contains 85% water, 70% of which can be exchanged, it induces lubrication according to the "liquid film" principle. In contrast, menisci contain only 74% water and are up to six times less permeable than cartilage. So it is not clear how much of the lubrication is usually attributed to the meniscus.

Imaging of meniscal lesions [11]

In the literature, numerous diagnostic radiological examinations have been described for the evaluation of meniscal lesions. However, magnetic resonance imaging (MRI) is the most accurate and least invasive method for the diagnosis of meniscal lesions. This technique has revolutionized knee imaging and has become the "gold standard" for meniscus imaging. It allows confirmation and characterization of the meniscal lesion, its type, extension, association with a cyst, meniscal extrusion, evaluation of cartilage and subchondral bone. The studies have shown excellent results regarding the sensitivity and specificity of MRI in the diagnosis of meniscal lesions. They allow the classification of different meniscal lesions, particularly in the early detection of grade I and grade II lesions in order to reduce the rate of unnecessary diagnostic arthroscopies.

Standard radiography :

Standard radiography is extremely limited in the evaluation of meniscal lesions, as menisci are not normally visualized with this type of examination. Standard radiography is therefore not useful in the investigation and diagnosis of meniscal lesions. Nevertheless, conventional knee radiography may be requested in case of doubtful diagnosis or differential diagnosis such as osteoarthritis, which frequently occurs at the same time as meniscal degeneration. Thus, this examination is recommended in cases of suspected meniscus injury in patients over 50 years of age, due to the frequent risk of associated osteoarthritis. A pinch in the line spacing of more than 50% or even a complete pinch may cast doubt on the reality of a possible symptomatic meniscal lesion.

X-rays can also remove unsuspected lesions, such as osteochondritis or foreign bodies. Finally, in the presence of a discoid meniscus, radiographs may show a relative enlargement of the compartment concerned, in this case most often the lateral compartment.

The radiography of the face and profile must be carried out in monopodal support, but also in incidence of schuss allowing to appreciate and compare the height of the interlines of the bearing zone compared to the contralateral side.

The radiography makes it possible to analyze :
- the quality of the bone structure
- the thickness of the femoro-tibial spaces
- densification of the internal or external tibial plateaus

Ultrasound :

Knee ultrasound is a very useful examination for the diagnosis of tendon injuries (patellar tendon, quadricipital tendon, crow's feet tendons) and peripheral ligament injuries (medial collateral ligament, lateral collateral ligament). Joint effusions (hydarthrosis or hemarthrosis) and cysts (communicating or not communicating with joint) are very well seen on ultrasound.

On the other hand, ultrasound is little used as a diagnostic tool for meniscal pathologies. It cannot examine the deep structures of the knee with great precision, and the accuracy of ultrasound depends on the skill of the radiologist (operator-dependent). The reliability of ultrasonography for the diagnosis of meniscus injuries is very diversely appreciated in the literature and does not seem satisfactory at present. It is therefore not a routine examination in meniscus imaging. Only meniscal cysts are easily diagnosed with a sensitivity of 97%, a specificity of 86% and a precision of 94%, and can possibly be punctured under ultrasound control.

Arthroscanner

Spiral acquisition allows to obtain multiplanar reconstructions of excellent quality with fine cuts of 0.5 mm.

Coronal, sagittal and even radial reconstructions allow the detection of cracks not visible on MRI, but also capsulo-meniscal disinsertions by passing the contrast medium between the meniscal wall and the peripheral capsule. This examination also allows a precise analysis of the cartilage of the femorotibial and patellofemoral joints with a precise mapping of the lesions. Arthroscanning is very little used in Anglo-Saxon countries, but remains a reference examination in the analysis of cartilage with meniscal lesions in Europe.

In the analysis of meniscal lesions, this test has a sensitivity and specificity between 86% and 100%. Arthroscanning of the knee is a safe technique that provides an accurate diagnosis in the identification of meniscus and cartilage injuries in patients who cannot be evaluated by MRI (Claustrophobia, Pace-maker) or in patients after surgery allowing the analysis of meniscus sutures and the condition of the cartilage covering the articular surfaces.

Magnetic resonance imaging

Magnetic resonance imaging (MRI) is the most accurate and least invasive method for diagnosing meniscal lesions. It is more accurate than physical examination and has influenced clinical practice and patient care by eliminating unnecessary diagnostic arthroscopies.

This technique has revolutionized knee imaging and has become the "gold standard" for meniscus imaging. Its advantages are the analysis in all planes of the meniscal lesion space, its excellent resolution by the different sequences allowing a very good soft tissue analysis. Its parametric character allows, depending on the sequences used, to privilege the visualization of a particular lesion or structure.

It allows to confirm and characterize the meniscal lesion, its type, its extension, its association with a cyst, meniscal extrusion, evaluation of cartilage and subchondral bone. From this fagon, MRI allows an accurate evaluation of the stability and probability of propagation of the fissure. It also makes it possible to determine whether or not the meniscal fissure is repairable or not in preoperative phase. [11]

a) Advantages and disadvantages of MRI :

The following sp_ntle. advantages:

MRI does not expose the patient to ionizing radiation. MRI does not routinely require intravenous administration of contrast material, the use of which is sometimes associated with adverse effects. MRI does not require manipulation of joints. MRI is painless and can be performed in less than 20 minutes.

MRI does not require the intra-articular injection of contrast material.radiographic iodized, unlike
arthroscan it. Arthrography with arthroscanner has been supplanted by MRI except for patients who are too large to fit in the MRI unit or for patients who have contraindications to MRI (e.g. intracranial aneurysm clips, orbital metallic foreign bodies or PACE MAKER, recent stents). MRI is also very useful for the diagnosis of residual or recurrent meniscus lesions after meniscus surgery. Its analysis

L_esjnconvénients_ou.contresÌndicat.ion.s_so_ntles.-s.uÌYants-:

MRI is limited in patients with claustrophobia, obese patients (weight over 170 kg) or who have a pace-maker. Its usefulness is also limited by the presence of artifacts created by nearby orthopedic equipment. Depending on the implant used, a variable amount of artifact is observable on MRI at the location of the fixation material. However, the use of non-ferromagnetic metals such as titanium has reduced the amount of artifact in the post-operative knee. Following the use of bioresorbable screws, artifacts interfering with the MRI study became much more limited. The additional advantage of bioresorbable screws is that all associated artifacts tend to decrease over time. The use of open MRI machines, as well as dedicated end units, decreased the number of patients for whom MRI cannot be used due to claustrophobia or obesity. For patients with definitive contraindications to MRI, computed tomography (CT) scan during an arthroscanner should be considered as the alternative imaging modality.

b) MRI technique

Low, medium and high field strength MRI machines (1, 1.5 or 3 Tesla) can all produce accurate diagnostic images to identify meniscal anomalies. For low field strength MRIs, the number of excitation sequences must be increased to obtain a correct meniscal image. This adjustment, however, increases the time required to form the images and thus the sequences, which in turn increases the risk of patient movement. Indeed, a small amount of movement can degrade the images, compromising the ability to diagnose meniscal lesions. [11]

A specific extremity coil antenna is used to optimize the signal-to-noise ratio. The sensitivity of detection of lesions of the medial meniscus is between 86 to 96% with a specificity of 84 to 94%. For the lateral meniscus, diagnostic sensitivity is 68-86% and specificity is 92%-98%. 11] Differences in sensitivity and specificity could be related to the sequences used, inter-observer variation, or sample size. Sensitivity for the detection of meniscal tears is generally higher for the internal meniscus regardless of the technique used. The MRI commonly used is a 1.5 tesla (T) MRI and produces high quality diagnostic images. There is little data in the literature comparing 1.5 T and 3.0 T MRI musculoskeletal imaging. It is expected that faster image acquisition at 3.0 T should result in more accurate imaging, or better diagnosis.

c) Protocols and imaging plan

The knee is generally positioned in extension with a slight external rotation to facilitate imaging of the anterior cruciate ligament (ACL).

High spatial resolution is necessary to show meniscal fissures.

This requires a field of view of about 22 cm (or less), a cut thickness of 3.3 mm (or less). A space of 0.3 mm is used between the imaging sections. An extremity coil is used to optimize the signal-to-noise ratio [11].

Images must be obtained in the three planes of sagittal, coronal and axial space.

Sagittal images are obtained with the knee in slight external rotation to allow imaging in the plane of the anterior cruciate ligament (indeed, meniscal and ligament injuries are frequently associated).

Several factors must be taken into account when optimizing imaging protocols. Imaging in all three planes is useful, however, not all sequences should be performed for all planes.

Usually, T1 sequences are performed in the sagittal pian, while T2-weighted sequences are performed successively in the 3 planes of space (sagittal, coronai and axial). Among the available sequences, it is necessary to distinguish between anatomical sequences and more pathological sequences. The meniscal structure and meniscal contours are better appreciated on proton density and T2-weighted sequences.

- so-called anatomical sequence: these are mainly T1-weighted and proton density weighted sequences. An MRI scan of the knee will almost systematically include a T1 sequence in the sagittal plane, thus making it possible to assess the state of the cruciate ligaments, the morphology of the menisci, the osteochondral structures, the extensor apparatus (patella, patellar tendon, quadriceps) and the joint cavity.

- So-called pathological sequences: these are sequences using fat signal suppression, whether STIR or T2 spin echo weighting sequences with specific fat signal suppression (T2 and T2 FSE Fat-Sat). This sequence is the reference for the analysis of intra-articular lesions: joint effusions, edematous infiltration, ligament or tendon rupture, bone contusion, subchondral bone edema, muscle injury, and especially meniscal lesions.

- There are other more specific sequences:

T1 Fat Sat Gadolinium sequence (T1-weighted sequence with fat signal suppression and intravenous gadolinium injection). This sequence has the advantage of being anatomical but also very sensitive on all inflammatory and/or vascularized structures.

T2 sequence (T2 gradient echo), this sequence is little used in the other joints (shoulder and ankle) and is sometimes used for the knee. Its main interest, apart from its very high sensitivity for the detection of meniscal fissures, consists mainly in the search for signs of chronic bleeding in the form of haemosiderin deposits, in the context of villo-nodular synovitis.

The most reliable MRI sequences for the meniscus are Proton Density Sequences (FSE) and T2 Fast Spin Echo T2 sequences but also Rho FSE Fat Sat sequences.

d) Normal meniscus MRI

A normal meniscus appears as a triangular low signal formation on the classical T1 and T2 weighted sequences or on the Fast-Spin Echo (FSE) sequences. The low signal is related to a lack of mobile protons within the normal meniscal fibrocartilage.

In children, a grade 2 signal is often seen in the posterior meniscal horns. This is considered normal and corresponds to the vascular system of a child's meniscus. This hypersignal disappears in adulthood.

e) Classification system for meniscal lesions

The MRI semiology of meniscal fissures is well codified. The use of the Stoller et Crues classification in 3 stages [11] has proven its reliability (sensitivity: 87 to 97%, specificity: 89 to 98%, reliability 88 to 95%. Only stage 3 abnormalities (linear hyper signal communicating with joint) should be retained as pathological.

This MRI classification was developed in correlation with a histological model. Areas of degenerative lesion show a hypersignal of variable intensity depending on the location and severity of the meniscus lesion. This classification excludes peripheral capsular disinsertions of the meniscus, which are considered non-articular.

Lesion... grade_1.

Grade 1 is a non-articular, focal or diffuse meniscus crack.

This finding correlates with early meniscal degeneration.

The terms myxoid degeneration or hyaline degeneration are used interchangeably to describe these lesions.

Injury.grade.2

Grade 2 is a horizontal linear hypersignal image in the body of the meniscus that extends to the lower surface of the meniscus without crossing it.

This abnormal signal is more extensive than in grade 1 but no cleavage or tear plane is present. Grade 2 is the progressive degeneration of Grade I. Patients are generally asymptomatic. The grade 2 signal can be of three types.

- Type 2A is a linear signal without contact with the articular surface.
- Type 2B is an abnormal signal in contact with one of the articular surfaces on a single cut.
- Type 2C is a very extensive signal but not in contact with the articular surface.

Lesiongrade_3

Grade 3 corresponds to an abnormal signal in the meniscus extending over a large part of the meniscus and communicating with at least one articular surface of the meniscus. Nevertheless, about 5% of grade 3 are intrameniscal fissures without any real meniscal cleavage. They may not be diagnosed in routine arthroscopy if the crack extension to the surface is not identified intraoperatively.

In addition to this description of lesions, there are two pathological criteria for meniscal lesions

These two criteria were established in MRI for the diagnosis of meniscal lesions. If no prior surgery has been performed on the meniscus, the diagnostic accuracy of meniscal lesions is more than 90% [11].

- Criterion 1: Corresponds to a signal alteration within the meniscus compatible with a crack, found on at least two consecutive cuts; this is the "Two-slice-touch rule" concept with a positive predictive value of 94% of meniscal fissures for the internal meniscus and 96% for the lateral meniscus. The positive predictive value was 55% and 36% for medial and lateral meniscal lesions when viewed on a single slice. The intensity of the abnormal signal must be in contact with an articular surface, either the upper surface or inside or at the end (free edge) of the meniscus. If contact with the articular surface appears on two or more consecutive images, the accuracy of the meniscus tear diagnosis increases.

- Criterion 2: focuses on the morphology of the meniscus. A thorough knowledge of normal meniscus MRI anatomy is required. Meniscal lesions are analyzed on both sagittal and coronai slice planes. Visualization of a meniscal fissure on these two planes of view reduces the rate of false positive diagnoses. However, some fissures at the meniscocapsular junction may be visualized on only one of the different slice planes.

<u>**3D Isotropy Turbo Spin-Echo MRI (3D Isotropy Turbo Spin-Echo MRI)**</u>

The 3D MRI in three dimensions with isotropic resolution has been developed, for the creation of multiplanar reformatted images, in order to obtain from an acquisition in a single slice plane, reconstructions in the other planes of space, or even in the axis of a structure defined as a ligament structure. In addition to the visualization of the structures in 2D and 3D, this technique also makes it possible to reduce the total duration of the MRI examination by a relative fagon. Furthermore, 3D MRI allows the visualization of small anatomical structures and can minimize the effect of partial volume due to its low section thickness. Finally, its field of study can cover the entire region studied without any free interval between the different slices. Thus, 3D MRI has received increasing attention in musculoskeletal imaging because most anatomical structures are small and oriented in variable directions, often oblique, especially in ACL imaging. Until recently, most isotropic 3D sequences were based on gradient-echo imaging, which has drawbacks such as increased risk of artifact and lack of contrast between normal and pathological tissue. Recently, the use of turbo-spin-echo sequences (TSE) has made it possible to acquire 3D isotopic images within an acceptable scan time. The knee joint is one of the most frequent applications of 3D isotopic sequences. The TSE sequence is considered as the best sequence for the evaluation of internal knee structures due to its high tissue contrast resolution. TSE sequences have diagnostic performance comparable to routine spin-echo MRI sequences, with respect to the overlying cartilage, menisci, ligaments and subchondral bone. Recent studies have shown that standardized TSE sequences even allow the detection of a larger number of meniscal lesions and in particular the early stages of osteoarthritis [11].

The discoid meniscus

Discoid meniscus is a meniscal dysplasia which causes the meniscus to occupy an excessive place in the inter-femoral- tibial space.
It is either complete or partial dysplasia. It is not an exceptional pathology in adults and its incidence is not specified in children, for whom few publications have been published. [12]

History :
External menisci of the discoid type have been known since Young's first description [13] in 1889. It was then an autopsy discovery, confirmed by the work of Kroiss [14] in 1910. Bristow [15] in 1927, very briefly reports a case. The first descriptions of clinical cases date from 1934 to 1936 [16,17,18,19,20].

It is noted that the external meniscus is more often affected than the internal meniscus, and bilateral involvement is classically described as rare: 5 to 20% of discoid menisci [12].

Pathogenesis :

No pathophysiological or pathogenic explanation for the occurrence of these abnormalities is considered to be very satisfactory [21]. The exact etiology of the discoid meniscus is unclear, and two main theories have been put forward: 1. the embryological theory: Smillie believes that these discoid menisci are linked to a halt in embryological development [22,23]: the discoid meniscus is the result of incomplete regression of the mesodermal blastoma, which normally begins to degenerate at 8 weeks of gestation [24]. 2. The second theory: Kaplan [25] contests this ethiopathogeny and believes that initially there is hypermobility of the posterior horn of the meniscus due to the absence of posterior tibial attachments (the menisco-tibial ligament) [26], this anomaly is responsible for abnormal movements with subluxation-reduction of this posterior segment during flexion-extension of the knee [25,22], these abnormal movements would be responsible for repetitive lesions of the meniscus which would then take a discoid form, thus hypertrophy and malformation would be acquired [25].

Positive diagnosis :

No clinical signs are evocative, but the discoid meniscus is a fragile meniscus so the patient may present a symptomatology made of interline pain, feeling of internal disturbance, cracking ...

Diagnosis, which was based on arthrography, is currently performed by MRI [27]. The references found in the literature, as far as ultrasonography is concerned, concern acquired meniscal lesions in adults [28-29].

In the work of Maeseneer et al. 30], the authors compared the contribution of MRI, arthrography and ultrasound and in the work of Maeseneer et al. exploration of the normal internal meniscus and in the diagnosis of capsulo-meniscal disinsertion. The contribution of ultrasound was found to be inferior to MRI not in the diagnosis of meniscal lesion, but in the diagnosis of capsulo-meniscal disinsertion.

In MRI, the diagnostic criteria for discoid meniscus are studied by several authors and are variable. According to Araki et al. [31], transverse diameter measured in the coronal plane (length) is the best diagnostic criterion and is greater than 14 mm when the meniscus is discoid. (Fig 1 and 2).

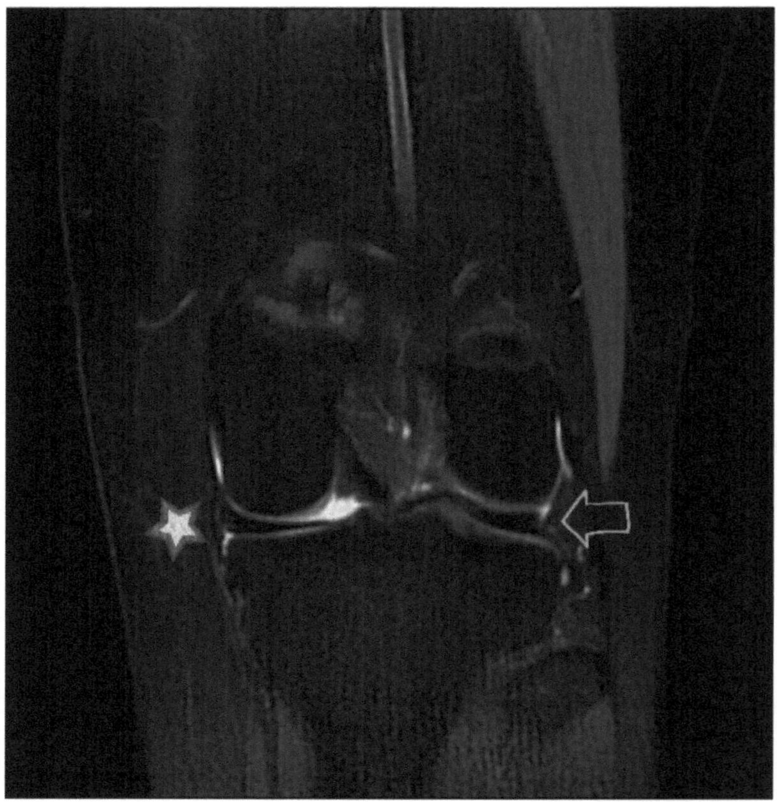

Figure 1: Magnetic resonance imaging (MRI) of a child's left knee in coronal section in DPFat-Sat sequence: enlarged external meniscus extending to the intercondylar notch, in hyposignal (arrow). Note the normal appearance of the internal meniscus (star).

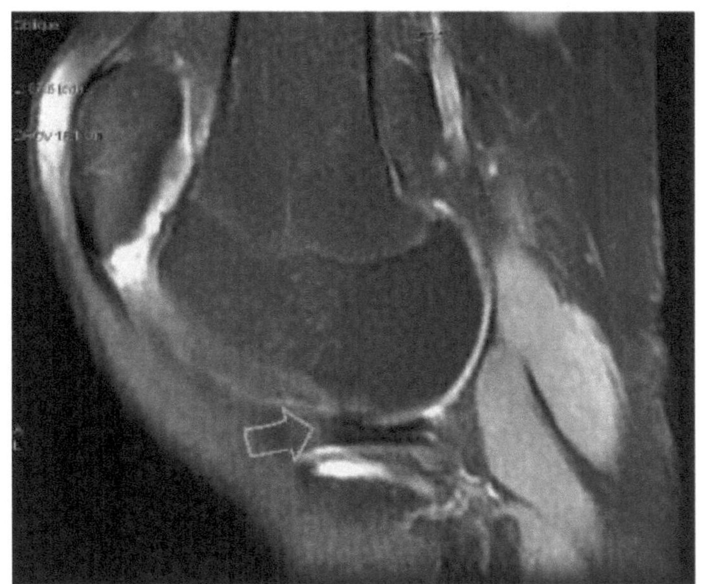

a

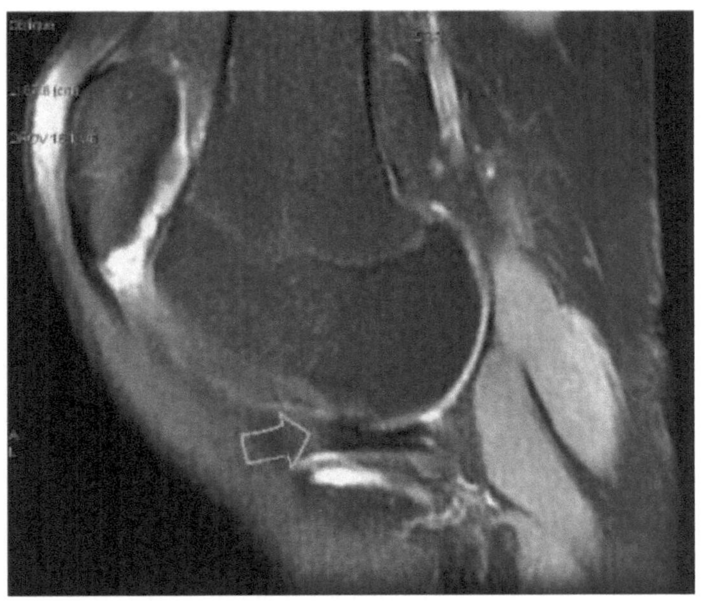

b

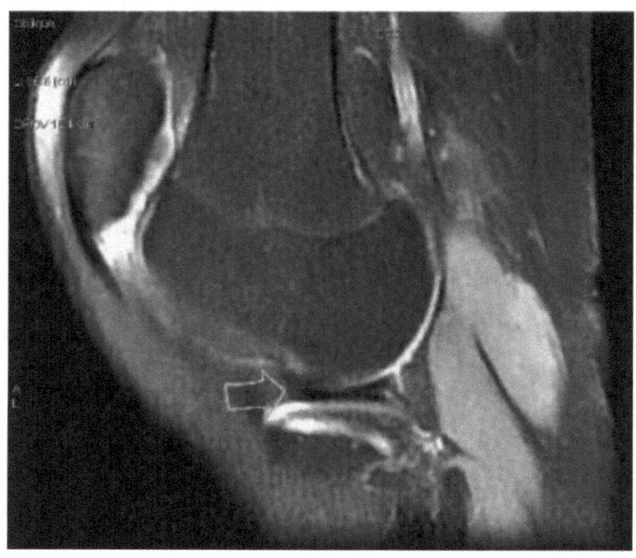

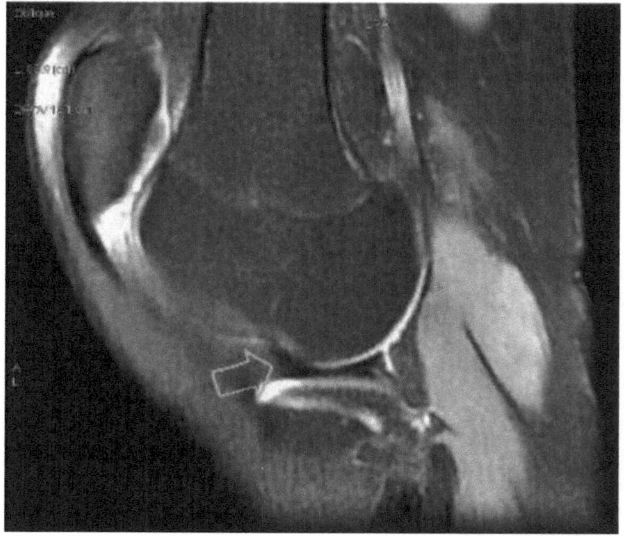

Figure 2 . (a,b,c,d) Magnetic resonance imaging (MRI) of a child's left knee in DPFat-Sat sequence sagittal slices passing through the external meniscus on 3 successive sagittal slices showing continuity between the anterior and posterior horn (arrows).

According to Stark et al. (13), the transverse diameter of the discoid meniscus averages 22.4 mm (ranging from 10.5 mm to 36.7 mm), and the thickness is 6 mm. Meniscal lesions are visible as a central hypersignal arriving or not arriving at the meniscal surface. [32]

Silverman and collar. 33], have associated criteria measured in both the sagittal and coronal planes: the meniscus is discoid when it is visible on 3 or more contiguous sagittal sections of 5 mm thickness showing continuity between the anterior and posterior horn, and when the difference in height between the pathological external meniscus and the normal internal meniscus is greater than 2 mm.

Somato and col. 34] took up all these elements and defined, in addition to the classical criteria, two other new criteria that they found more sensitive:
- the ratio between the minimum meniscal length and the maximum tibial length measured in the coronal plane. It must be greater than or equal to 20%.
- the ratio between the sum of the thickness of the anterior and posterior horns of the meniscus with the largest meniscal diameter measured in the sagittal plane. It must be greater than or equal to 75%.

We note that in children, the presence of an intra-meniscal band in hyper T2 signal is very characteristic. It may be related to a traumatic lesion that is frequent in these patients [35] or to a fluid degeneration classically described in these children [12].

The classification :

A- External discoid meniscus :

In his 1948 article, Smillie [23] proposed the first classification essentially related to the thickness of the meniscus, he described 3 types:

- Primitive or massive

- Infantile, or almost normal

- Intermediate between the two previous ones.

Since Watanabe et al [36], the classification has been based on the proportion of surface area covered by the tibial plateau and comprises 3 types (it actually combines the classifications of Smilie [23] and Kaplan [25]):

- The complete type, in the shape of a disc thinner in the center
- Incomplete, half-moon type, with central edge and convex or concave.
- The hypermobile or "Wrisberg" type, without posterior tibial insertion.

Completed by Monleau and others in 1998, it includes 4 types : (Fig.3)

- Complete when the entire lateral tibial surface is covered, and constitutes 70-80%.

- Incomplete when this surface is partially covered, constitutes 10 to 26%.

- Wrisberg" type when the discoid meniscus lacks its posterior bony attachment on the tibial plateau and is inserted on the posterolateral part of the medial condyle in continuity with the

"Wrisberg" ligament, resulting in a hypermobile meniscus, rarely reaching 8%.

- Ring-shaped when the meniscus has a completely circular appearance but is open in the center and constitutes 4 to 5% . [37-38-39]

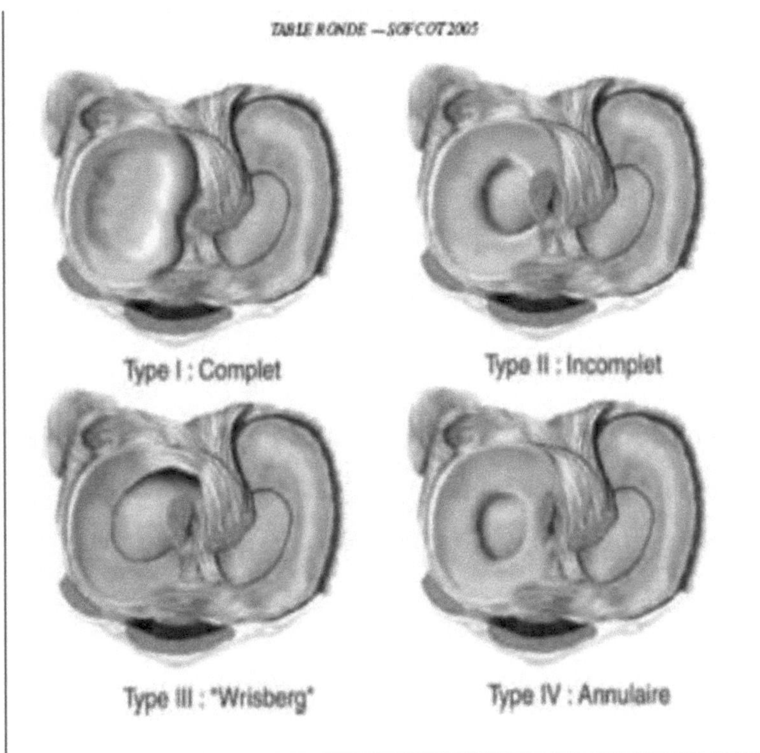

Figure 3: Watanabe classification completed by Monleau in 1998

B- Discoid internal meniscus :

The classification of discoid internal menisci has never been proposed in the literature, probably because published cases are scattered and rare. There seem to be only 3 types:

- Complete, massive, similar to Smillie type 1;

- Incomplete, with concave free edge, like Smillie type 3;

- In disc perforated in its center.

<u>Treatment :</u>

The surgical treatment of discoid menisci has been discussed repeatedly, and several therapeutic modalities have been proposed: First of all, therapeutic abstention, which has always been the rule in the case of asymptomatic discoid menisci [40]. The radiological discovery of a discoid meniscus does not impose its surgical treatment. Only symptomatic discoid menisci will be subject to surgery [40-41].

Surgical treatment by total or partial meniscectomy (Figures 4 and 5) is justified only if the discoid meniscus has a lesion [42-43].

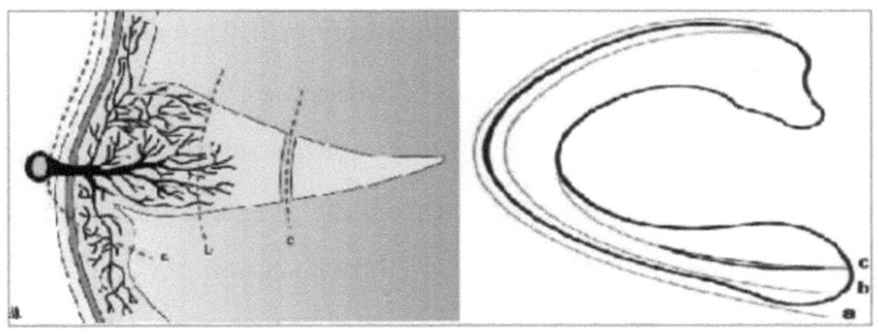

Fig 4 : Different types of meniscectomy sections

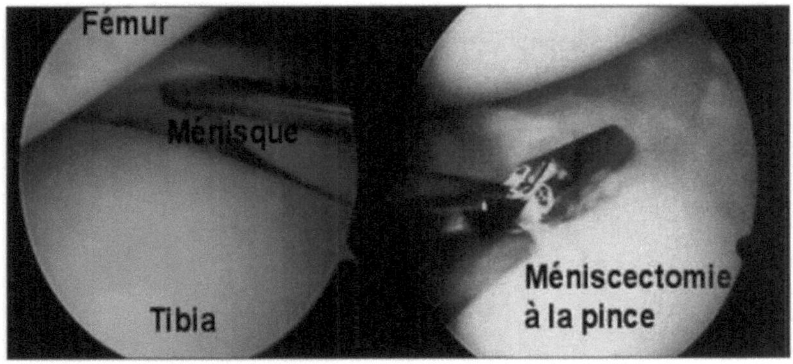

Fig 5 : Partial internal meniscectomy per-arthroscopic

Total meniscectomy is rarely necessary. Proposed by Kaplan [25] and defended by Kurosaka [44] . It can sometimes still be indicated for major peripheral lesions with associated complex lesions, respecting if possible 3 to 4 mm of the meniscal wall. Watanabe type III often requires a total meniscectomy more or less extended to the anterior segment [45].

Meniscectomy is most often performed under arthroscopy, which has revolutionized knee surgery in terms of its diagnostic and therapeutic aspects, allowing a precise description of the lesions, especially type III wrisberg [21], and a rapid and healthy recovery [46]. However, it can be converted into arthrotomy [47] in case of difficulties. Ikeuchi and other authors [48] recommend a mini-arthrotomy for the anterior part, which also makes it possible to suture the retinaculum to tighten the capsule and thus prevent the lateral instability favoured by resection of the meniscal volume located between the cartilage surfaces.

Adachi et al. described five cases of discoid meniscus lesions treated by meniscoplasty and suturing. These five cases showed good clinical results, including four excellent results after more than two years of follow-up [49]. Ahn et al. in 23 patients (28 knees) treated with meniscoplasty and meniscal repair, found 21 excellent results with an average follow-up time of 51 months [50].

List of figures

Figure 1: Magnetic resonance imaging (MRI) of the left knee in coronal section in DPFat-Sat sequence: enlarged external meniscus extending to the intercondylar notch, in hyposignal (arrow). Note the normal appearance of the medial meniscus (star).

Figure 2. (a,b,c,d) Magnetic resonance imaging (MRI) of the left knee in sagittal sections in DPFat-Sat sequence passing through the external meniscus on 3 successive sagittal sections showing the continuity between the anterior and posterior horn (arrows).

Figure 3: Watanabe classification completed by Monleau in 1998

Figure 4: Different types of meniscectomy sections

Figure 5: Partial internal meniscectomy per-arthroscopic

References

1. Gardner E, O'Rahilly R. The early development of the knee joint in staged human embryos. J Anat 1968;102:289-99.

2. Arnoczky SP, Warren RF. Microvasculature of the human meniscus. Am J Sports Med 1982;10:90-5.

3. DeHaven KE. The role of the meniscus. In: Ewing JW, editor. Articular cartilage and knee joint function. Basic science and arthroscopy. New York: Raven Press; 1990. p. 103-15.

4. Fithian DC, Kelly MA, Mow VC. Material properties and structure-function relationships in the menisci. Clin Orthop 1990;252:19-31.

5. Mow VC, Holmes MH, Lai WM. Fluid transport and mechanical properties of articular cartilage: a review. J Biomech 1984;17:377-94.

6. Fithian DC, Kelly MA, Mow VC. Material properties and structure-function relationships in the menisci. Clin Orthop 1990;252:19-31.

7. Arnoczky SP, Adams ME, DeHaven KE, Eyre DR, Mow VC. Meniscus. In: Woo SL, Buckwalter JA, editors. Injury and repair of the musculoskeletal soft tissue. Park Ridge: AAOS. 1988. p. 487-537.

8. Mow VC, Kuei SC, Lai WM, Armstrong CG. Biphasic creep and stress relaxation of articular cartilage in compression. Theory and experiments. J Biomech Engin 1980;102:73-84.

9. Fairbank TJ. Knee joint changes after meniscectomy. J Bone Joint Surg Br 1948;30:664-70.

10. Dejour H, Bonnin M, Neyret P. In: Anterior cruciate deficient knee stability in monopodal stance: the influence of the posterior slope of the tibial plateau, of the medial meniscus and of the posteromedial corner. Proceedings of the 4th Congress of the european society of knee surgery and arthroscopy. 1990. p. 445.

11. Lefevre N, meniscus imaging. http://www.chirurgiedusport.com/

12. Bennani Smirès CH, Benjalloun A, Dadi- Benmoussa F, Hamdouch M, Zeghari

H, Zouaoui A. Magnetic resonance imaging and discoid meniscus in children. J Radiol 1998;79:861-4.

13. YOUNG RB. The external semilunar cartilage as a complete disc. In: Cleland J, MacKay JY, Young RB eds. Memoirs and Memoranda in Anatomy. London, England: Williams and Norgate; 1889:179.

14. KROISS, F. The injuries of the intercondylar cartilages of the knee joint and their connections. Beitr. z. klin, Cbir 66: 598, 1910.

15. BRISTOW, W. R. Anatomical variation of the semilunar cartilage. Proc. Roy. Soc. Med., 21: 241, 1927.

16. DUNN, N. Observations on some injuries of the knee joint. Lancet, I: 1267 1934.

17. FINDER, J. G. Discoid external semilunar cartilage a cause of internal derangement of the knee. J. Bone Joint Surg,16: 804. 1934.

18. BELL-JONES, E. The discoid or congenital abnormality of the interarticular fibrocartilage of the knee joint. Liverpool Med.Chir. J., 43:78,1935.

19. JAROSCHY, W. The sliding meniscus lateralis genu as a cause of the fasting knee. Beitr. z. Klin. Chir., 161:139,1935.

20. FISHER, A.G.T. The disc-shaped external semilunar cartilage. Brit. M.J., I: 688, 1936.

21. JACQUES RODINEAU, PROJECTING GERARD. Anatomical anomalies and sports pathology, 2004 p: 137-144.

22. ANDRE FRANK, T AIT SI SELMI, HERNI DORFMAN. Société franose d'arthroscopie 2006: Congenital meniscus lesions. J-F, Kempf, P.Clavert.

23. SMILLIE I. The congenital discoid meniscus. J Bone Joint Surg (Br), 1948, 30, 671-682.

24. GRYNFLETT. Développement de l'articulation du genou chez l'homme, Montpellier medical, 1904,25,613-655.

25. KAPLAN EB. Discoid lateral meniscus of the knee joint; nature, mechanism, and operative treatment. J Bone Joint Surg (Am), 1957,39,77-87

26. SILVERMAN JM, MINK JH, DEUTSCH AL. Discoid menisci of the knee: MR imaging appearance. Radiology 1989; 173: 351-4.

27. Manco LG, Lozman J, Coleman NP, Kvanaugh JH, Bilfield BS, Dougherty J. Non invasive evaluation of knee meniscal tears: preliminary comparison of MR imaging and CT. Radiology 1987;163: 727-30.

28. Fracr RP. Ultrasound in acute and chronic knee injury. Radiol Clin North Am 1999;37:797-829.

29. Azzoni R, Cabitza P. Is there a role for sonography in the diagnosis of tears of the knee menisci? J Clin Ultrasound 2002;30: 472-6.

30. De Maeseneer M, Lenchik L, Satrok M, Pedowitz R, Trudell D, Resnick D. Normal and abnormal medial meniscocapsular structures: MRI imaging and sonography in cadavers? Am J Roentgenol 1998; 171:969-76.

31. Araki Y, Yamamoto H, Nakamura H, Tsukaguchi I. MR diagnosis of discoid lateral menisci of the knee. Eur J Radiol 1994;18:92-5.

32. Stark JE, Siegel MJ, Weinberger E, Shaw DWW. Discoid menisci in children: MR features. J Comput Assist Tomogr 1995; 19:608-11.

33. Silverman JM, Mink JH, Deutsch AL. Discoid menisci of the knee: MR imaging appearance. Radiology 1989;173:351-4.

34. Somato N, Kozuma M, Tokuhisa T, Kobayshi K. Diagnosis of discoid lateral meniscus of the knee on MR imaging. MRI 2002;20:59-64.

35. Stark JE, Siegel MJ, Weinberger E, Shaw DWW. Discoid menisci in children: MR features. J Comput Assist Tomogr 1995; 19:608-11.

36. WATANABE M, TAKEDA S, IKEUCHI H. Atlas of arthroscopy. Berlin. Springer-Verlag, 1979. 1998, 14, 502-504.

37. MONLEAU J, LEON A, CUGAT R, BALLESTER J. Ring-shaped lateral meniscus. Arthroscopy,

38. RAO PS, RAO SK, PAUL R. Clinical, radiologic and arthroscopic assessment of discoid lateral meniscus. Arthroscopy, 2001, 17, 275-277.

39. HAYASHI LK, YAMAGA H. IDA K. MIURA T. Arthroscopic meniscectomy for discoid lateral meniscus in children. J Bone Joint Surg (Am), 1988, 70, 14951500.

40. ANDRISH J. The diagnosis and management of meniscus injuries in the skeletally immature athlete. Operatives techniques in sport medicine, 1998, 6, 186-196.

41. MARK D MILLER, KEVIN D PLANCHER, RICHARD F. Surgical atlas of

sports medicine, 2005 p,18-21.

42. Locker B,Hulet C, Vielpeau C. Traumatic lesions of the menisci of the knee. Editions techniques-EMC- Appareil locomoteur.14-084-A,192

43. W. K.AUGE AND C.C KAEDING. Bilateral medial discoid menisci with extensive intrasubstance cleavage: MRI and arthroscopic correlation, 1994.

44. KUROSAKA M, YOSHIA S, ONHO Y. HIROATAKAK. Lateral discoid menisectomy. 20 years follow-up. presented at the American academy of orthopedic surgery meeting, 1987 January ; san Francisco, Etats unis.

45. AICHROTH P, PATEL D, MARX C. Congenital discoid lateral meniscus. A follow-up study and evolution of management. J Bone Joint Surg (Br), 1991, 73, 932-936.

46. David C. Neuschwander; J. BONE JOINT SURG. 1992, VOL 74-A, 1186/1190.

47. ANDRE FRANK, T AIT SI SELMI, HERNI DORFMAN. Société franose d'arthroscopie 2006: Congenital meniscus lesions. J-F, Kempf, P.Clavert.

48. IKEUCHI H. Arthroscopic treatment of the discoid lateral meniscus. Technique and long-term results. Clin Orthop Relat Res, 1982, 167, 19-28,

49. Adachi N, Ochi M, Uchio Y, Kuriwaka M, Shinomiya R. Torn discoid lateral meniscus treated using partial central meniscectomy and suture of the peripheral tear. Arthroscopy 2004;20:536-42.

50. Ahn JH, Lee SH, Yoo JC, Lee YS, Ha HC. Arthroscopic partial meniscectomy with repair of the peripheral tear for symptomatic discoid lateral meniscus in children: results of minimum 2 years of follow-up. Arthroscopy 2008;24:888- 98.

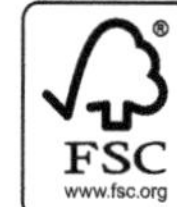